by Larry Terkel
One of America's Most Experienced Meditation Teachers

INCLUDES
A Meditation Session (Mp3 download)
Larry leads you through a complete meditation session.

A GREAT TOOL FOR GETTING STARTED!

email: **meditation@SecretstoMeditation.com**
for your free download.

How to
meditate
Secrets to the Easiest and Most Effective
Meditation Technique

carrot
seed
PUBLISHING

Carrot Seed Publishing LLC
44 West Case Dr.
Hudson, OH 44236

info@carrotseedpublishing.com
www.carrotseedpublishing.com

Book designed by Ari Terkel

ISBN 978-0-9834115-4-3

Library of Congress Control Number: 2011907450
1. Self-Help / Meditation. 2. Self-Help / Spiritual.
3. Health & Fitness / Yoga. 4. Health & Fitness / Healthy Living.

Printed in the United States of America
10 9 8 7 6 5 4 3 2 1

SecretstoMeditation.com
MeditationPlus.net

Acknowledgments:

First, I want to thank my family. My son, Ari, urged me to share what I have learned in over 40 years of meditation. His wife, Alicia, along with my daughter, Marni, and son, David, all jumped on the encouragement bandwagon. With her love, support and enthusiasm, my wife, Susan, taught me how to write. As the author of many books and my co-author for *Small Change* (Tarcher/Penguin), Susan told me I was ready to write this alone. It was scary at first, but I love her for that confidence and insight.

Special thanks go to my astute and excellent editor, Lorna Greenberg, and all of the staff at Carrot Seed Publishing.

Additional thanks go to the teachers and students at the Spiritual Life Society including Matt and Gennie Lerner, Robb Blain, Carson Heiner, Lisa Thiel and Nichole Miller. Also, to my friend and early spiritual partner, Erik Holmlin, thank you for sharing the teachings you brought home from Nepal. And thank you Marilyn Wise for your feedback and support.

Finally, I have been blessed to have had incredible and inspiring teachers in my life. Thank you to Father Dan Berrigan, Rabbi Rudolf Rosenthal, Swami Satchidananda, Rabbi Joseph Gelberman, Brother David Pendergast, Teruchi Swami, Dr. Joseph Politella, Pir Vilayat Inayat Khan, Swami Vishnu Devananda, Satya Sai Baba, B.K.S. Iyengar, Baba Ram Das, Lilias Folan, Yogi Amrit Desai, Swami Rama, Swami Muktananda, Shantji and Swami Bawra.

Dedicated to the memory of my grandfather and first spiritual mentor,

George Klein

Table of Contents

In 1969, the Cornell University Interfaith Religion Department, led by the famous anti-war activist, Father Dan Berrigan, sponsored a weekend workshop on comparative religion.

The three presenters were: Swami Satchidananda, Rabbi Joseph Gelberman and Brother David Pendergast. Their goal was to discuss their various traditions, and to explore their similarities. It proved to be a weekend that changed my life.

I was enthralled with all three men. Adopted at birth, I was raised in a Jewish family, with very little exposure to other religions. I would also say that the Judaism I was exposed to, while religious, was not particularly spiritual. Oh, I did go to Hebrew School twice a week, but my studies there were confined to learning to read Hebrew and preparing for my Bar Mitzvah at the age of thirteen.

Rabbi Gelberman was nothing like the rabbi I knew from our temple. There was excitement in his voice when he talked about his tradition. He described a Judaism that encouraged questions – questions of each other, questions of ourselves, questions of God. Instead of presenting a Judaism that was pickled in the past, he presented a live and vibrant relationship with the Divine that was continually developing and unfolding.

All I knew about Hinduism was that its many gods seemed the antithesis of Judaism's monotheism. But Swami Satchidananda presented the unity of Divinity that underlies Hinduism's apparent diversity, with each of the individual gods symbolizing specific aspects of Divinity itself.

Brother David Pendergast was a Benedictine monk from the Christian "contemplative" movement. He presented the possibility that through a personal relationship with Jesus Christ, we could be led into a deeper relationship with the Divine realm.

Actually, what I remember most is not what anyone specifically said. What I remember is the impression they left – an impression of joy, of genuine caring, of wisdom and of love. Their smiles spoke volumes. Here were living examples of people whose paths had been different, yet who had arrived at the same spiritually-fulfilled place.

I came away with one other impression. I learned that what they had in common was a technique found in each of their traditions. Each had practiced meditation extensively. For each, it was meditation that had brought them harmony, and meditation had deepened their relationship with the Divine. Meditation had brought them insights into themselves, into their religion and into the world around them. Meditation had brought them a measure of peace, clarity, wisdom and love.

I remember leaving the weekend thinking I wanted some of what they had found. I wanted some of that peace and clarity. I wanted some of that wisdom, some of that love. But I left not knowing how to get it. Their teachings on how to meditate seemed vague. It was not at all clear to me how to actually "do" it.

I knew, however, that meditation was something I wanted to do, so I set myself a goal. I would learn how to meditate. I would read books on meditation. I would explore Transcendental Meditation, which the Maharishi Mahesh Yogi had brought to the United States a few years earlier. I would travel to India and study with masters from one end of the country to the other. And I would begin what was to become the most significant and rewarding habit of my life – the practice of meditating for 10 to 30 minutes, *every single day.*

It is over 40 years later. I have now spent over 5,000 hours of my life in meditation, which is the equivalent of seven months (without sleep) of solid meditation, seven months of peace and quiet, seven months of listening and paying attention, seven months of cultivating perspective and helping me overcome the challenges in my life.

In 2004, I wrote *Small Change; It's the Little Things in Life that Make a BIG Difference* (Tarcher/Penguin). It was a finalist for a National Books for a Better Life Award. It was reprinted by M.J. Fine and featured at the front of Barnes and Noble for several years. It has been published in Japan, France, Italy and Korea. I have been interviewed all over the United States and one of the most frequent questions I am asked is: "What has been the most powerful small change you ever made, the one that has had the greatest impact on your life?" Without hesitation, I say, "Meditation."

Meditation has helped me succeed in business by helping me find solutions to the many problems that arise. Meditation has been a constant throughout over 40 years of marriage to my delightful wife and fellow meditator, Susan. Meditation has provided both of us continuous teachings on the power and importance of love. Meditation has brought us the patience needed to raise three active, outgoing children. Meditation has given us the perspective that their way in the world does not have to be the same as ours. Meditation provided us with the vision to establish the Spiritual Life Society, a yoga, meditation, and spiritual center we founded in a historic church we acquired in 1978, in our town of Hudson, Ohio. Meditation remains the core of my teachings there. And meditation is what has helped me maintain balance in my work, family life, leisure activities and spiritual pursuits. Indeed, without meditation, it would have been easy to lose that balance.

You, too, can have similar benefits – and more – without struggling through the years it took me to learn the simple, yet powerful, techniques that await you in this book. The teachings that follow are based on my experience and my practice. They do not come from other books. They come from my life and my experience, from meditating and teaching meditation. I personally attest to everything I am about to share with you.

I promise that if you follow these simple instructions, and find at least 10 minutes each day to practice the meditation I'm offering, your life will change dramatically. You will become clearer, healthier, wiser, less stressed, more peaceful, more creative and more loving. You will be able to bring into your life exactly what you need to know, whenever you need to know it.

How can I be so positive? Because only 10 minutes per day will add up to 60 hours of meditation in a year. That's 60 hours spent in peace, 60 hours spent pursuing clarity, 60 hours spent cultivating wisdom, perspective, creativity and love. Those 60 hours, as much as it sounds, is less than one percent of your time, yet it will make the other 99.4% immeasurably better.

What a deal!

There is an ancient saying, "When the student is ready the Master appears." Most people take it at face value, and are waiting for the Master to appear. They are waiting for the perfect relationship to bring them the perfect love they seek. They are waiting for new medications to heal whatever ails them. They are waiting for a sign from God that God exists and will bless them with whatever they want or need. They are waiting for the "Master to appear."

Alas, the wisdom in the saying is not the "Master appearing." The wisdom is in the student "being ready" – ready to change habits, ready to explore something new, ready to discover the wisdom, faith and love that *already* resides in you and is waiting for you to release.

What makes people "ready?" The bad news is that it is usually suffering that makes a person ready. For many of you, it is probably suffering, in some form or another, that brought you to this page in this book. Something in your life is not going well. Perhaps you are one of the 60 million people in the United States who do not get enough sleep, and have heard that meditation can help with that problem. Perhaps you are suffering from anxiety and stress, with side effects such as high blood pressure, anger or substance abuse, and have heard that meditation can help you overcome these problems. Or perhaps you suffer from depression, feelings of loneliness and unworthiness, and have heard meditation can help you as well.

Suffering is a message that it is time to change, time to do something different to escape from the pain and discomfort of your life. And yes, meditation will help.

There is, however, another way to get ready, though most people do not avail themselves of this path. That is to decide that even though life is going pretty well, it could always be better. You may have heard that meditation will not only cure problems but will make life that much more enjoyable, that meditation can elevate your life to even higher levels of satisfaction. Perhaps you are an athlete who would like to excel at your sport. Perhaps you are a student and would like to learn more effectively and efficiently. Perhaps you are pregnant and want to give your baby a peaceful, low-stress environment in which to develop. Perhaps you are simply searching for greater meaning and to bring a positive, spiritual perspective into your life. Meditation will do these things and more.

Are you "ready?" Are you ready to alleviate that suffering? Are you ready to elevate your life? I am confident that the meditation practice you learn from this book will change your life as much as it has changed mine, and that it will bring you all the joy, happiness, wisdom, creativity, peace and love that you seek – and deserve.

Enjoy your journey!

Allow me to begin by explaining why I call the meditation technique I am about to teach you the easiest and most effective for you to practice.

To do so I need to give you an understanding of the meditation techniques that sages have practiced for thousands of years. Generally speaking, there are two basic approaches, one stemming from the Buddhist tradition and the other from the Hindu tradition. (Don't worry, you won't have to become Buddhist or Hindu to meditate effectively. I'm just giving you some background.)

The Buddhist system centers on a free-flowing technique called *vipassana,* which can be translated into "insight," and is taught in the United States under the names "insight meditation" or, as I will refer to it, "mindfulness meditation." In contrast, the Hindu system is more focused, usually involving concentration on a mantra – a word or phrase that brings you into oneness with its meaning and vibration.

In mindfulness meditation the idea is to become a witness to your thoughts, feelings, sensations and breathing. You become a witness to what is going on both inside your body and mind, as well as outside. The idea is to cultivate a sense of detachment, understanding that what you are witnessing is normal but in everyday life we are too busy to pay attention to it. By seeing your thoughts and feelings for what they are, just thoughts, just feelings, you take away their power to carry you into directions you may not want to go. Under ideal circumstances, mindfulness meditation calms our fears and anxieties that may be attached to those thoughts or feelings.

Furthermore, while mindfulness meditation helps develop detachment, it also builds up your sense of being a witness. Who is this witness that has thoughts and feelings but isn't those thoughts and feelings? It tunes you into what is sometimes called the "higher self" or "true self." Alternatively, it may be called "higher consciousness," the ability to transcend the lower consciousness of your thoughts and feelings.

Let's be clear. I love mindfulness meditation. You will see many of its principles included in the technique you are about to learn. The problem I have always had with it is that I don't find it easy. It doesn't give me an anchor. I know that the witness is supposed to be my anchor but my mind can be too loud, too distracted and too uncooperative. Also, studies have shown that in some people, witnessing their thoughts and feelings can actually be counter-productive without professional guidance. People who have suffered major loss or trauma may not have the skill to detach from such powerful thoughts, fears, or feelings.

The other major meditation technique involves giving the mind something specific to focus on. By focusing the mind, other thoughts can subside and the mind can become calm, relaxed and quiet. The classic technique utilizes a mantra – a word or phrase to repeat over and over in your mind. This is the technique made popular by Maharishi Mahesh Yogi known as TM, or Transcendental Meditation. Dr. Herbert Benson, the Harvard researcher, uses a simplified version of mantra meditation to elicit what he calls the *Relaxation Response.*

With its repetitive chants and prayers, it could be argued that Christianity and Judaism tend to utilize the focused, mantra system as a way to train the mind and connect it to divine teachings and insight. However, neither mindfulness nor mantra meditation need be considered attached to any specific religion. Yes, there are religious forms of both. But the techniques themselves can be used with or without religious connections.

In some ways, mantra meditation is considered easier than mindfulness since you know exactly what you're supposed to be doing. It's not as free-flow as mindfulness. You know when you feel you are meditating and when you're not. The difficulty associated with mantra meditation is the complication (or expense) of figuring out what mantra to use.

The technique you are about to learn combines the best of both approaches. My students like to call it *Meditation Plus.* It is mantra meditation **Plus** mindfulness. I demystify the process of choosing or obtaining your mantra. I treat the mantra as a thought or vibration to be mindful of, to be witnessed and even enjoyed. I offer you the option of choosing a mantra that fully supports your religious tradition, no matter which one that is. Or you can choose a mantra without religious connotations, opting instead for one with more generic or universal appeal.

By showing you how easy it is to choose or receive your mantra, by sharing with you secrets I have picked up along the way to help anchor your practice, it will be ever so easy to know what you are doing and why. The secrets incorporate your tongue and your eyes, and draw on your experience with swings and duets. They will convince you that *Meditation Plus* is the easiest and most accessible way to meditate.

Then there's the issue of "most effective." It's fair to ask: most effective for what? This is where my practical business approach enters the picture. I say that something is effective when it helps you solve some of the many problems you face in your life. Let's look at how *Meditation Plus* does this.

Most meditation practices will succeed in reducing stress and inducing a state of relaxation, at least for the time you are doing it. During meditation the breath calms, the muscles relax, the heart beats slower and blood pressure lowers. We become more peaceful and more centered. Then what? Do you return to the stresses and tensions of your life with your blood pressure returning to elevated levels? Was the meditation just an enjoyable respite from which you must return to the problems of your life?

Some schools teach just that. You meditate for the joy of the meditation, nothing more, nothing less. The idea is to get addicted to that peace. Spend more and more of your time there. Let the rest of your life, including your responsibilities, fall away like illusions. Only the meditative state counts as the true reality. It becomes the definition of enlightenment, and that enlightenment becomes the goal of your meditation.

I have always had a problem with that teaching. I think it's great if you want to become a monk and spend your days meditating in a monastery at the top of a mountain searching for enlightenment. But that was never my goal. I wanted a family. I wanted to help others. I wanted to challenge myself to find creative solutions to the problems that human life presents. I practice meditation because it aids me in pursuing those goals, not as a goal in itself.

I will teach you how to use the meditative state you achieve in your practice to find creative solutions to the problems you face in your life. Relationships, work, illness and injury all bring with them problems and challenges that require wisdom and perspective if we want to be able to claim the satisfaction, joy, happiness and peace we all want to achieve.

I know some teachers will say you are chasing an illusion. After you solve one problem another will arise. Success is fleeting. Only God is real. Well I happen to love the ancient teaching that says, "Trust in God but tie up your camel." I teach my students to develop a personal relationship with the Divine. I teach that meditation provides both a *peek* experience and a *peak* experience of the Divine realm. But you shouldn't take away from that experience that because the spiritual is great and magnificent, the material world is just a bad dream. It's not spiritual *or* material. It's spiritual *and* material. This world teaches us about peace, love, joy, triumph and success just as it teaches us about anger, fear, suffering and loss. We are here to learn. The world is our teacher. Meditation can be incredibly effective in facilitating that learning.

That is why I will teach you how to capitalize on the meditative state you achieve by following it with a period of clear creative thinking. After you have spent at least 10 minutes meditating, after you have achieved the state of detached witness, after the mantra has brought your mind into a focused and consciously chosen vibrational state, I will show you how to direct that clarity and creativity towards the problems in your life. I will teach you how to use it to generate options and choices so you can choose which choice is wisest to pursue. You will want to have pen and paper at your side when you meditate to take notes. You will want to capture your insights. You will want to use them to change or improve your everyday life.

I encounter many students in my classes and workshops who tell me they used to meditate and stopped because they didn't think it was doing enough to warrant the investment of time. Their biggest question for me is: what has sustained my over 40 years of daily meditation? What makes me want to sit everyday? My answer has always been: it's not the meditation, it's the insight it gives me that I'm addicted to. My wife feels the same way. We couldn't have written the books we have without it. I couldn't have managed my various businesses without it. Our relationship wouldn't be as deep. Our health wouldn't be as good. I look forward every day to seeing what my meditation will produce for me that day. It may be an idea. It may be an insight. It may be a solution to a problem. It may only be the day's to-do list. But that to-do list will have things on it that a normal to-do list won't. It may include tell my children how much I love them. It may include apologizing to my wife for something I said or did. It may involve a change to my diet. Whatever it is, I continue to be amazed at the wisdom I receive.

It is that thinking, that problem solving, that clarity, that enhanced creativity that is the real plus in this *Meditation Plus* technique. That is the plus that you will be motivated to achieve. That is the plus that will provide solutions for the problems causing your tension in the first place and, when combined with the relaxation produced by the meditation itself, will really reduce the stress in your life. That is the plus that will reduce your blood pressure and enable you to sleep better at night. That is the plus that makes the *Meditation Plus* technique you are about to learn so effective.

Your mind is an incredible tool.
In addition to regulating all of
the muscles and organs of your
body, it does two other things
extremely well. One is that it
stores memories. It files away
into your memory banks all
of the experiences you have
ever had, all the pain, suffering,
mistakes and disappointments,
and all the joys, triumphs,
insights and accomplishments.

Sadly, scientific studies have confirmed that we tend to hold negative memories closer to the front of the file than positive memories. As the saying goes, "We remember the tears far longer than the laughter."

What the mind also does is generate thoughts and ideas. It is like an electric generator pumping out wave after wave of energy for you to use to power your lights and electrical appliances. You choose how to use the power it provides. Like an electric generator, the brain pumps out wave after wave of thoughts and ideas. You choose how to use the thoughts and ideas generated by your mind, as well.

This generator analogy brings us to a major issue regarding meditation in general. Most teachers and books say that the goal of meditation is to quiet the mind, to bring the mind to a profound level of stillness, to turn off the generator as much as possible. This goal sounds great until you sit down to meditate and your mind refuses to cooperate. It refuses to be quiet, and when it does get quiet, the boredom can be excruciating. Your mind offers a million different things it would rather be doing, and when that occurs, you begin to think that meditating is hopeless. Nor does it help to see your teacher – or a photo of your teacher – sitting serenely blissful in front of you, which may only convince you that they have a skill you will never attain.

Wrong! Very, very wrong! First of all, know that your teacher is still thinking, even when it appears as if he or she isn't. It is not the "thinking" that needs to stop for you to be "meditating." It is your *relationship* with your "thinking" that needs to change for you to be "meditating." So let's get this straight. The first secret you need to know is that meditation is not about "not thinking." In fact, some meditation techniques, such as mindfulness meditation, are all about observing what the mind is thinking.

Here is what determines the difference between thinking and meditating. "Who is in charge?" In normal life your thoughts take charge. Something happens, and you react in the way your mind tells you to react. One day your daughter is late from school and your mind dismisses it, immediately assuming she stopped at a friend's home. Another day she is late again and you jump to the conclusion that something terrible has happened. Perhaps you heard a story on the morning news about a child kidnapped from a mall. Your mind takes you in one direction or another and you dutifully follow.

When, however, we take time to examine the thoughts our mind is presenting, we realize there are many possibilities. We can choose which thoughts to follow, but most of the time we don't avail ourselves of those choices. It's as if we are on autopilot. We drive to work the same way everyday. How much of

the drive do you remember, unless something out of the ordi-
nary happens to grab your attention?

In meditation, we take a different approach to our thinking
and change the subject to the object. Instead of dutifully following our mind's lead, we step back and observe our mind and
its thoughts, as if from a third-person perspective. We see our
thoughts for what they are – just thoughts. Like the trees you
see as a green blur as you drive past in a car, thoughts can
pass through your mind in a flash. But then you find a tree to
focus on, and follow it until it's out of sight. During meditation,
your thoughts are like those trees. Your mind presents them,
but you get to choose which one to focus upon.

Meditation is the process of defusing your thoughts of their
power. You become a witness, a partner, a second party to the
process of thinking. You are no longer the servant or victim of
your thoughts. You become both a spectator and a voluntary
participant. Meditation makes you a person-who-has-thoughts
instead of a thinking-person. That may not sound like much – a
person-who-has-thoughts versus a thinking-person – but the
difference is profound. Meditation puts the power of your mind
at your disposal, and with that power, that consciousness, you
can make a big difference in your life – physically, mentally,
emotionally and spiritually.

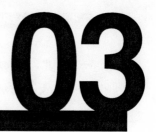

03

You may or may not know the word "mantra." It has become common as a word or phrase that expresses a guiding principle for you to follow in seeking a successful outcome for your actions.

A golfer might adopt "Keep my head down" as a mantra. By thinking it before swinging, you give your mind a plan to follow with the expectation that if followed, the ball will hit the target. Nike offers another example of a mantra in its marketing slogan "Just do it."

In spiritual communities and secret societies throughout history, mantras have been ascribed many mysterious powers. Witchcraft is said to derive power from secret incantations that can create spells and affect circumstances. Great spiritual masters are said to have used mantras to become able to see the future, read someone's mind, materialize objects or levitate their bodies off the ground. In Sanskrit, powers such as these are called *siddhis,* and are said to be bestowed upon only the most earnest and diligent practitioners.

I am fascinated by the subject of mantras. The intriguing claims that surround them are what attracted me to meditation over 40 years ago. Like a lens focusing a beam of light into the power of a laser, could a mantra focus our minds to amazing power as well?

In this chapter, and the next two chapters, I attempt to pull back the curtain, reveal the mantra's source of power and demystify the mantra meditation practice. My hope is that you will not need the enticement of secret powers and other-worldly gifts to motivate you to meditate. Instead, your motivation will be based on evidence, logic and realistic expectations. I promise that you will experience results no less magical than those ancient claims of the power of mantras. The behind-the-scene understanding you gain will not diminish the amazement you experience. It will enhance it.

Let's begin.

A mantra is simply a word or phrase that you use as the focus of your meditation. On one level, a mantra is just a thought, one of the trees you choose to focus on in the forest. However, it is not just any thought. It is a word or phrase with two defining characteristics.

First, a mantra contains an important message or meaning. That message may convey a sense of higher power, such as your religious tradition's name for the Divine. It may convey some aspect of the Divine, such as Divine Spirit or Divine Love. A mantra may also be a word or phrase that conveys some desirable attribute you would like to bring into your life, such as healing, love, peace or wisdom. It could express gratitude for blessings you have received or blessings you hope to bring into your life. The meaning or message, however, must represent something important you want to attract into your life.

Second, like any word, a mantra, when spoken, has a sound, a vibration that can be heard and felt. It is as if you can feel the meaning of the word – feel the power of its message. Think of a tuning fork used for tuning a musical instrument. You listen to its vibration, then tune the string on your guitar accordingly. When the string is in tune, it vibrates in harmony with the tuning fork. Since your mind and body are your instruments, it's important to keep them in tune with the qualities and values you hold most dear. This is what your mantra can do for you. It brings you into harmony with its higher message, with the quality and meaning it represents, with the vibration it evokes.

Returning to the message of Chapter Two, remember that meditation is not about stopping thoughts, but rather, about bringing thoughts into perspective. The mantra – a specific, meaningful thought, with a specific vibrational component – has the power to help you become a witness to your thoughts. It has the power to help you experience the "Self" in you, as one-who-has-thoughts, not simply as one-who-thinks. The mantra puts itself – and all other thoughts – into clarity. Will other thoughts compete with and disturb your focus on the mantra? Of course they will! That's the job your mind has. But, everytime you return to the mantra, with its message and its vibration, you will be reminded of who you are and who's really in charge of your mind.

Let me close this chapter with a personal story that illustrates the power of a mantra. It also serves as a warning to choose your mantra wisely. Know what the meaning is. Know what the vibration conveys.

When I began this journey in 1969, most of my guidance came from Hindu swamis and Indian teachers. The mantras offered were in strange languages, such as Sanskrit. I was told that it wasn't necessary to understand the meaning of the mantra, that each mantra had been perfected by masters of the past, and through its vibration, the mantra's power was available to me. I was also taught that the most powerful mantra was the sound OM, with its phonetic spelling as AUM forming the equivalent of three syllables, ah-oh-mmmmmm.

I was young, enthusiastic and determined to go right to the top of the mantra list. I began an earnest, twice-daily meditation practice using the mantra OM. When I returned from India in 1971, and began my career as an engineer, I brought that OM meditation practice home with me. I would rise early in the morning to do yoga, then meditate for 30 minutes before going to work. When I returned home from work I would meditate again, for another 30 minutes, before having dinner and spending the evening with my wife. My plan was to use the morning practice to get me ready for the long workday, and the evening practice to cleanse me of work issues so I could enjoy my evening with Susan. That's not exactly what happened.

As time went on, I became more and more attached to my meditation practice. It was what I wanted to do more than just about anything else. If we were invited to a friend's home on the weekend, I didn't want to go. If we were invited out to dinner and a movie, I didn't want to go. I wanted to meditate and bask in the peace that meditation brought me.

My obsessive desire to meditate continued for three years, until a close friend came to visit. Erik had just spent two years in Katmandu, studying meditation with Buddhist monks and teachers with the esteemed title of *Lama*. We began comparing our experiences and our practices, and I told him I was using the mantra OM. Erik said five words to me that I remember as if it was yesterday. He said, "Lamas say, OM... monk trip!"

In a flash I realized the effect the mantra was having on me. OM is a reclusive vibration. The teaching is great for monasteries and caves. It is not for an active, western family life. I decided to leave OM for the monks and seek a new mantra and a new approach to meditation. I began using the technique I am sharing with you in this book. I want you to know the meaning of the mantra you use. The ancient masters knew what their words meant. I want you to know what effect you can expect your mantra to have on you and your life. You need to tune your instrument to the music you want it to play. Tune it wisely. Tune it carefully. Tune it to embrace the power you desire and deserve.

Levitation is the ability to lift one's physical body off the ground with little effort. It is one of those powers, *siddhis*, that has been sought by yogis for thousands of years. Most people consider levitation impossible. When a magician levitates an assistant we assume it's an illusion, with some secret trick that the audience simply can't see.

I love to explain to my yoga students that levitation is actually quite easy. Almost everyone can do it. In fact, almost everyone has done it at some time in life. You can levitate, too. How? Just sit on a swing. I know, you're disappointed at how easy I am making this, but take a moment to think about it.

On a swing you channel your effort to lift the entire weight of your body off the ground. You literally experience the exhilaration of momentary weightlessness without anyone's help. You don't have to kick hard, and you don't have to exert much effort, but you do have to know the secret: You have to *kick at the right time.* By leaning and kicking at the right time, each kick will allow you to swing higher and higher, until either fear, or the limit of the swing's rope, bring you back down to earth.

Think about how almost everything in life follows the same rhythmic, back and forth motion of a swing. Breathing follows a rhythm of inhaling and exhaling. Hearts beat, then rest. Eating and sleeping have a rhythm. The world swings between day and night, summer and winter, fast and slow, exciting and uneventful. Emotions peak and subside. Thoughts come and go. Health gets interrupted by illness or injury. The economy fluctuates. Relationships swing from dramatic to peaceful. Happiness rises and falls.

Everything about life ebbs and flows because life and all its components are, in effect, swings. We are born to swing, and it is human nature to want to elevate our swings and our lives to higher and higher levels. The history of civilization can be seen as a swing that, despite the wars and setbacks, continues to climb higher and higher. Wouldn't it be great if we could elevate our personal lives, elevate our health, wealth and happiness, to higher and higher levels?

Here's the good news. With meditation you can do just that. The secret power at work on the swing and the secret power at work in the *Meditation Plus* technique you are about to learn, is the power of harmony. Yes, you must kick when sitting on a swing and it takes some effort to kick. But think about this. The effort you need to exert on a swing to lift you off the ground is far less than you would exert if you were trying to lift a barbell as heavy as your body. On a swing, harmony multiplies the small effort required to lift your weight. Harmony multiplies the timing of a gentle kick into the power of a weightlifter.

Here's another example of the power of harmony. Your car is stuck in a ditch. How can you get it out? If you gun the gas and apply maximum effort, giving the tires as much speed and power as possible, you might expect to propel the car out of the ditch. Right? Sorry. All that effort may just dig a deeper ditch!

The best strategy is to get your car to rock back and forth, *in harmony* with the contour of the ditch. It is the timing of going from forward to reverse – the effort applied *with harmony* – the rocking back and forth instead of gunning the gas that has the power – the real power – to elevate a 2000-pound car out of a ditch. Effort alone won't work. Visualizing the car out of the ditch won't work. Swinging back and forth, in harmony, will provide the power you need.

Being in rhythm – in harmony – requires less effort, but brings results far greater than you can imagine. Engineers have a name for this phenomenon. They call it *harmonic resonance.* In fact, the power of harmonic resonance is recognized by scientists as *one of the most powerful forces in the universe.*

You will learn how to put the power of harmony to work in your meditation practice. You will learn how to get all the elements of *Meditation Plus* working together, in harmony with each other, to help you achieve the results you seek.

That harmony begins with a two-syllable mantra. I have found that two-syllable mantras are the easiest and most powerful to use. Why only two syllables? Because your breath consists of two syllables – an inhale and an exhale. The inhale is the acquisition phase that brings oxygen into your body. The exhale is the letting-go phase that eliminates the by-products of your respiration. The inhale energizes. The exhale relaxes.

Your breath follows the movement of a swing. The inhale is your backward motion, pulling the swing back, pulling the breath in. The exhale is your forward motion, letting the swing fly forward and up, letting your breath fly out.

In the next chapter you will learn how to receive your personal mantra – the perfect mantra for you to work with at this moment in your life. You won't need to pay thousands of dollars to a Maharishi, or travel to India to have some master give you a mantra. You will know that it is safe and you will understand what makes its two-syllables so powerful.

When we get to the step-by-step meditation instructions in Chapters Nine through Twelve, you will see that every step is aimed at achieving harmony – harmony in your body, harmony in your mind, harmony with others in your life, harmony with the world around you, harmony with the Divine. The harmony begins with the breath and embodies the vibration of the mantra, but it ends up connecting you to the realm of the Divine. It is easier and more fun to dance when you can hear the beat and feel the rhythm of the music. It is easier and more enjoyable to meditate when you can harmonize your mantra with your breath.

Remember this secret, and apply it to every aspect of your life: **Harmony multiplies effort, helping you swing higher in everything you do.**

Many ancient Eastern writings emphasize the value of a personal teacher, or guru, who can guide you on your spiritual journey. They describe the guru-disciple relationship as magical, ordained by the Divine, and one of the greatest karmic gifts you can earn after lifetimes of struggle.

They say that upon meeting your guru you recognize each other immediately, and acknowledge your divine connection with one another. You will feel as if you had always known each other, as if your guru had always been watching over you, knows everything about you, and can see through you to the core of your being.

This guru-disciple bond is purported to be nothing short of mystical, your spiritual destiny manifested in a flash of absolute clarity. There have certainly been many times when I have longed for just such a moment. In 1970/71, I traveled the length and breadth of India, meeting masters and searching for that mystical connection. The list of masters whose presence I have experienced is long and impressive. Some were famous, and universally recognized as great gurus. Others were obscure, yet clearly in possession of great spiritual power and wisdom.

Here's my take, and it harkens back to this book's introduction, where I talked about "When the student is ready the Master appears." Remember that I discussed my belief that the wisdom of that saying is "when the student is ready," and not "the master appears." Well, I believe that there are many masters, many teachers who can guide you on your spiritual path. I no longer believe there is only one master for each student. In some circles, this statement – that you can have many gurus – may be considered blasphemous, so let me explain.

I believe it is important to consider the original context in which a religious scripture has been written in order to extract its wisdom. I believe the scriptures must be interpreted. Imagine the Buddha in a garden, teaching his students. He sees a drunk falling off the path to his left. The Buddha interrupts his teaching and yells to the drunk, "Go right." His students write down that the Buddha said, "Go right." A few minutes later the same drunk is falling off the path to the right and the Buddha yells, "Go left." This time his students write that the Buddha said, "Go left." Anyone reading the students' notes will see that the Buddha contradicted himself by offering advice to go in two different directions. The only way to extract the Buddha's true instruction is to know the original context.

In ancient days access to teachings and teachers was limited. With no printing press, the only books were those copied by hand. Most teaching was verbal, handed down from teacher to student. There were no airplanes to whisk you away to distant lands in a few hours. To find an accessible teacher who possessed the knowledge you were seeking was indeed magical. The teachings could only be received by a relatively small number of students and, as I said earlier, those students had to be "ready." Because teachers weren't readily accessible, their teachings were treated like secrets. The few students who received them would have easily felt "chosen." No wonder the ancient literature praises the blessings of the guru-disciple relationship.

Times have changed. Information is shared instantly all over the world, at the speed of the Internet. Mass-produced books have turned "secrets" into general knowledge. Masters can "appear" at the touch of a few finger clicks.

Would you like to know what really happened to me on that trip in 1970? My first teacher was Swami Satchidananda, one of the three speakers I met at Cornell University the year before. We traveled and lived with him for three weeks at the beginning of our trip. I was even more enthralled than when I first met him. Wisdom seemed to pour forth from him effortlessly and consistently. He seemed to understand me so well. I could have described how I felt in the same magical words as the ancient literature. I have great memories from our time together. Many of his teachings changed my life dramatically. He gave me a mantra. He wanted to give me a spiritual name. He seemed to assume he was to be my guru for life.

I guess you could say I flinched. Either I wasn't quite "ready" or I wasn't quite convinced. It was too early in my journey to commit. I still had the whole country of India to check out. Maybe you could say I was a spoiled American who wanted to do some comparison shopping before buying. I didn't want to jump at the first choice, and felt I could return even more committed, if no other master could touch me like Swami Satchidananda.

As I went on to meet other teachers, I quickly began to feel skeptical. Each master seemed to use the same metaphors to answer the same difficult questions. Each invited me to become a disciple. Each tried to convince me to stay on his ashram and learn from him directly. Each began to sound just like Swami Satchidananda. He was the first to tell me that my guru search was like digging three-foot deep wells all over my property in an attempt to find water. His advice was to stay and dig deeply in one spot. The first time I heard that teaching I was impressed, but when five teachers in a row gave the same teaching as a reason to stay with him, I became a little jaded.

Soon, however, my disappointment in not capturing the magic that the ancient books had described, began to be replaced by a different understanding. I began to realize that each teacher, each master, each guru, was giving me something I needed. Each had his own personality. Each gave me a slightly different slant on what I was trying to learn. Each succeeded in broadening my understanding and my perspective. What might have become a journey of frustration became a journey of incredible good fortune. It was a blessing to be exposed to so much wisdom, and given so many powerful examples to follow, and in some cases, not to follow.

What does all this have to do with the subject of how you can receive your personal mantra? The answer is a lot, because in the ancient literature, mantras have been treated as mystically as finding your guru. Receiving a mantra is described as a direct transmission from guru to disciple. Receiving a mantra is supposed to carry the energy of your "enlightened" guru. The analogy is that it takes a fully charged battery to transmit sufficient energy to charge your dead battery.

Here's the contradiction found within the systems usually presented. At the same time that the teachings extol your magic relationship with the guru and the mantra, they teach – quite clearly – that the guru is ultimately to be found inside of you, and that your personal mantra resonates within you, as well.

My over 40 years of meditating and teaching meditation have shown that you do not need to have anyone else tell you what mantra you should use, or what mantra you need. You can heed the suggestions of a teacher you respect. But let's be honest. Many popular teachers in this country have proven to be less than perfect masters, including Bhagwan Shree Rajneesh,

Swami Rama, and Yogi Amrit Desai. I have met them all. Their teachings were impressive. They were all charismatic. Their followers were enthralled. But behind the scenes, one of them struggled with drugs, the others struggled with sexual promiscuity and the abuse of vulnerable disciples.

Given the imperfection of even "near-perfect" masters, why turn over your future, your decision-making to them? Yes, listen to their advice. Learn from their teachings. In the end, however, it is your life, and your life is defined by the choices you make. When you give up that responsibility (a word I teach literally as the ability to respond) to someone else, you become vulnerable. You have been given a discriminating mind. Use it. Listen to it. Make your own mistakes. Don't let someone else make them for you, leaving you to bear the consequences.

Let's discuss one more issue while we're on the topic of both gurus and personal mantras. That issue is the cost. By claiming to have the secret mantra you need, and describing the tremendous benefits and value you will receive from that mantra, teachers are attempting to justify the price you will have to pay. These teachers can sound like snake oil sellers, claiming meditation will cure all your problems and even bring about world peace. Of course, that mantra and the meditation skill that goes with it, are so valuable you will have to pay dearly to receive it. They even justify the high price by saying that the more you pay, the more you will value it, and the more committed you will be to meditating.

Now that I have unloaded a few of my prejudices, I want to add that I am not saying that what these gurus and teachers sell is valueless. I am saying that when the pitch sounds too good to be true, approach with caution. If you can afford it, try it. If you respect the opinion of someone else who has tried it, consider it. Just be realistic about yourself, your resources and the claims they promise to deliver. And remember, the ultimate teacher is within you.

My mantra meditation system does not rely on me or, for that matter, anyone else, giving you or selling you a mantra. Instead, consider your mantra to be a gift from the guru within, from the power of your own mind, from the world at large or from the circumstances you find yourself in. You can even consider it a gift bestowed upon you directly from the Divine. Its source is for you to decide. Of course, I will make suggestions to help you find your mantra. I will even offer you choices. But once you understand the system I teach, you will know that you are not limited by my suggestions. You will have the knowledge and the confidence to choose the mantra that's right for you. You will be "in on the secret."

I do offer you one guarantee – that every suggestion I offer you is a mantra I have personally worked with. I know that each of the mantras I offer is safe and I know that each is highly effective. If you believe that a mantra should come from someone who has already infused energy into it, then know that I have done so with each mantra I suggest.

So, how are you going to receive your personal mantra? You are going to receive your mantra from the sound of your breath. Yes, the sound of your own breathing. Breath is life, and life is a Divine gift. Breath gives life to every cell of your body. Your breath, your life, has a message for you, a message that it whispers in your ear – approximately 20,000 times each day! When you sit quietly and listen, you will hear its message, you will hear your mantra. Your mantra is formed by the two syllables of your breath, by the inhale and by the exhale. First listen for it. Then discern what it is saying. Sound hard? Let's try an example.

Some Eastern traditions teach that the sound of the breath is the Sanskrit word, *So-Hum*. Listen to your breathing for a moment. Can you hear the inhale whispering "So" and the exhale whispering "Hum?" One translation of this mantra is, "All that is…is." Another is, "Everything is Divine," or "God is everything." *So-Hum* is a message of amazement for all that is around us. I like to think of it as the "Wow" mantra, because it tunes you in to wonder, and carries the vibration of "Wow." *So-Hum* reminds you not to get lost in your petty problems, but rather to see the bigger picture, to remember your blessings, to be thankful for what you have and not dwell on what you don't have. *So-Hum* remains one of my favorite mantras.

Fortunately, *So-Hum* is not the only word or message you can hear your breath whispering. Another great mantra Westerners can relate to is *Amen,* (Ah-Men) a reminder that our life is a blessing. *Amen* is a statement of gratitude offered to the Divine. *Amen* carries with it a vibration of appreciation, a message of thankfulness for all we have been given, and all that we hope to receive.

Two other powerful Sanskrit mantras you can hear in your breath are *Sat-Nam,* a message and vibration of truthfulness, and *Shanti,* the Sanskrit word for peace. *Sat* means truth, and *Nam* means name, so *Sat-Nam* is often translated as, "Truth is God's name." This mantra reminds us to choose truth, to live truthfully and to strive for what is right. *Shanti,* being both the word and vibration of peace, reminds us to choose peace, and strive for peace – both inside ourselves and in the world around us.

You may hear a mantra that is common within your religious tradition. Some of the most magical words in all religions have two syllables, which I believe is not a coincidence. Indeed, some of the most powerful mantras are names we ascribe to the Divine. Note that the word *Divine* itself is two syllables, a wonderful mantra in itself, and I can assure you it carries a powerful vibration. It reminds you that all of life is Divine, that within each of us is the Divine spark of life itself.

In Judaism, the name for the Divine is *Yah-Weh,* a name that is never meant to be spoken aloud, but that mystical Judaism teaches can be heard in the sound of our breath. In Islam, *Allah* is another two-syllable name for the Divine, and can be readily discerned in the breaths we take. In Christianity, *Jesus* and *Mary* have two syllables. In Hinduism, most manifestations of the Divine have names and vibrations that are two syllables: *Brahma, Shiva, Vishnu, Krishna* and *Rama* are some of the Hindu mantras I have used. Each represents an attribute of the Divine, with its own personality and its own vibration.

Finally, English has several powerful two-syllable words, with distinct vibrations. Words such as *loving, healing* and *blessing* each make great choices for a mantra as they can be easily heard as a message your breath is whispering to you. I have also had great results with the mantra, *patience.* It is two syllables and is a powerful reminder that often, patience is what is needed in life. This mantra has helped me slow down and adjust my expectations – when slowing down and adjusting them were what I needed at the time. You will find a longer list of mantras for you to choose at the back of the book, including many more from the Judeo-Christian tradition.

Take a few minutes now to relax and listen to your breath. What do you hear your breath whispering when you listen? What message is the world trying to give you at this time in your life? What do you think you need to learn? What should you be remembering? What vibration, what pitch, what note or key do you want to tune your instrument to so you can play the music of your life as harmoniously as possible?

Let's turn to a common question that many meditators ask me about mantras. Can you change your mantra after you have been using one for a while? There is no hard and fast rule. I answer by saying of course you can change your mantra. Circumstances in your life can change and what you need can change with it. The teaching I give is the same parable that I was told in India by gurus encouraging me to be their disciple. If you dig three-foot wells all over your property you are not likely to find water. You must dig deeply in one spot.

It is important not to jump from mantra to mantra. Decide what makes sense for you now, and stick with it until the message that comes through your meditation is that it is time to change. If a different mantra seems to be interfering, seems to be getting louder and louder, as if the Divine is trying to get your attention, by all means, change. Just don't change frivolously. Dive in deeply to reap the rewards you deserve, and then move on.

What I hope you have learned from this chapter is that receiving your mantra is a combination of what you hear your breath saying, what the world is saying to you through your life's circumstances, what the Divine is encouraging you to become, and what you know you need to hear. Listen to your breath, then choose a mantra. Make it a collaboration with the Divine, or with the world or with your inner Guru. Resist the need to have someone else tell you what mantra you need. Your inner self already knows. Trust yourself. Trust the message of your breath. Then play your tune with confidence.

That brings me to one final point on the subject of mantras. The issue involves whether to tell others what mantra you are using. It relates to an old saying, "One should not cast pearls before swine." You run the risk of a negative comment stealing your confidence and trust. My advice is to be very careful with who you give that power.

Now, it's time to sit.

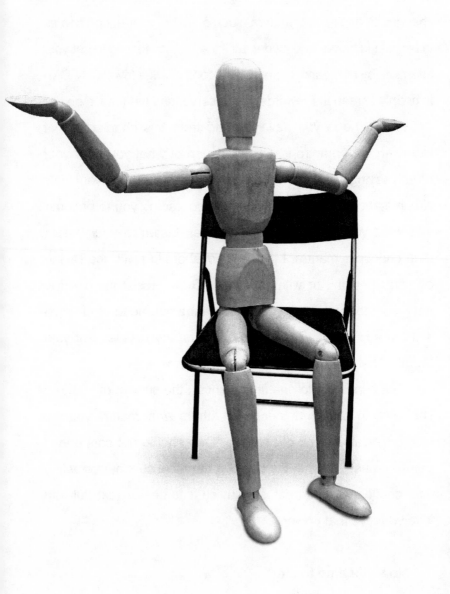

In the next three chapters you will learn how, where and when to sit for meditation. Before we get to any details, let's be clear. My primary teaching on how, where and when to sit for meditation is: Meditate anyway, anywhere, and anytime that you can. Now that I have said that – and I intend to repeat it many times – let's begin with your choices on how to sit.

We're beginning with how to sit because how you sit may determine where and when you meditate. There are two primary goals here: comfort and alertness. If your body is uncomfortable, the discomfort will be distracting, and it will be difficult to focus on your meditation. On the other hand, if you are too comfortable – perhaps curled up in your bed, or lying back in a soft reclining chair – you may not be alert enough to focus on your meditation. The challenge is to find a happy medium that maximizes both comfort and alertness.

Remember, I said you could meditate anyway you can. Some people can meditate while walking. There are even techniques designed for walking meditations. They capitalize on the high level of alertness associated with walking, and make awareness of your sensations the focus of the meditation. Mindfulness meditation works particularly well as a walking meditation technique.

Some people can meditate in bed. If you are disabled or bedridden due to injury or illness, bed may be your only alternative. Comfort will be maximized, but the challenge will be to maintain a level of alertness that keeps your brain from drifting into the lower brainwaves associated with sleep. Some suggestions are to remove the pillow and lie flat on your back, or draw your legs up into a crossed-legged position while lying on your back. Neither will be quite as comfortable as your favorite sleep position, but that is the idea. Trade off some comfort to gain alertness.

This brings us to sitting. For the reason above – the desire to maximize comfort and alertness – sitting is the recommended position as long as your body is capable. You can sit on the floor, sit in a chair or sit up in bed.

Let's look first at how to maintain alertness in any comfortable, seated position. Remember being in school, after too little sleep, with a teacher lecturing in a monotone on a subject that didn't interest you? What position did your body assume? Didn't you slump in the chair, round your back, lean your head back against the back of the chair or flop it forward onto your desk? Would you say you were alert?

Now remember how you sat in class when you had enough sleep, the subject was interesting, and the teacher was energetic and excited? You sat up straight. Your head was unsupported. You sat forward in your chair. You were interested, engaged and alert.

Alertness goes hand in hand with a straight back and an unsupported head that is balanced over your shoulders, not drooping forward or back, ready to nod off at any moment. This is your goal: to be able to sit up straight, your head unsupported, but still be as comfortable as possible, whether in a bed, in a chair or on the floor.

There's no reason why sitting up in bed can't meet the criteria of comfort and alertness. The key is a straight back and a balanced, unsupported head. Prop yourself up with a pillow in the lower back to straighten and lift your spine while keeping your head away from the wall or backboard. Your legs can be straight as long as the pillow keeps your back from rounding over too much. If you can, draw your legs up into a cross-legged position. After all, what's the difference between cross-legged on the floor and cross-legged in bed? It's the same position, and cross-legged on a mattress can be far more comfortable than on the hard floor. You don't get points for being macho here. You earn your points by meditating, and cross-legged in bed can be a great way to do it. You have my permission.

Enjoy.

Sitting in a chair is often the best choice for beginning meditators. Just remember, you want your back to be as straight and upright as possible so that you can remain alert. So if you choose to use your favorite soft chair, which can be a great place to start, you don't want to slouch or lie back in a reclining position. Like sitting up in bed, placing a pillow behind your lower back will support your spine in a more upright position.

Another option I have used is to sit cross-legged in that comfy chair, assuming it is wide enough to accommodate your knees. You may find you can sit quite comfortably and upright there, but if necessary, add a pillow for lower back support. This is how I meditate on an airplane, if the seat next to me is empty and I can put up the armrest to spread my knees.

Another chair option is to sit in a regular straight-backed chair. Again, the goal is to be as upright as possible. You can use a lumbar cushion to support your back or move forward on the chair. If you sit almost at the front edge, with your tailbone tilted slightly up in back, you will find that your lumbar curve will be supported in its natural position. Your spine and your head will be vertical and comfortable.

By the way, this is a better way to work at your computer as well. It's also a better way to eat. If you round your back while eating you are compressing your stomach and digestive organs. One of the easiest ways to prevent indigestion and heartburn is to move forward on your chair and sit up straighter.

Finally, there's the classic position pictured in books showing a monk, or yogi, sitting on the floor in a cross-legged position. Again, the challenge here is to be both comfortable and upright. Stiff hips and legs, for example, will make the process of crossing your legs uncomfortable after a few minutes. Because it takes vigilance and muscular effort to maintain a straight back, slouching over is a constant temptation.

This discussion of sitting comfortable and upright brings me to the topic of yoga. I am a yoga teacher as well as a meditation teacher. Yoga is great for preparing your body for meditation. Practicing the poses in yoga, called *asanas,* can enable you to open and restore your body to its natural, straight, properly aligned position. In fact, the ancient, classical teaching is that asanas are practiced *primarily* so that one can sit in meditation without the distractions caused by the body's discomfort. This goal has been lost to some extent in the West, where physical yoga is taught as a goal in itself. Many people here are attracted to the health benefits of a fit and flexible body, and that's to be applauded. My point is that too few are motivated to practice yoga in order to sit comfortably and pursue the even greater benefits that meditation has to offer.

Those who do study yoga will learn a number of sitting poses that help to straighten the back. One of the ultimate and elusive goals is to sit in the full lotus position, called *padmasana.* This is the classic pose which brings both feet onto the thighs, with both knees resting on the floor. I need to be honest here, and tell you that it took me eight years of practicing yoga *daily* to finally sit comfortably in *padmasana.* My advice, therefore, is to avoid rushing lotus, and instead meditate in a position that does not compromise your comfort.

I like to joke by telling my students that sitting in lotus is not a prerequisite for enlightenment. In fact, you will find that being honest and realistic about your limits will bring you closer to enlightenment than the false pride of showing off. I have already given you permission to sit on a chair or even sit up in bed. Do what's best for you.

The way to cheat and still sit cross-legged on the floor is to use a thick (4-6") pillow, or a folded blanket. If you can lift your buttocks sufficiently, it will feel as though you are sitting on the front edge of a chair. It will help bring your lumbar into alignment, straighten your back, and bring comfort to your crossed legs. Pillows made specifically for this purpose are call *zafus.* There are also meditation benches that accomplish the same goal by tilting your pelvis and lifting your spine while sitting on your knees. These can be quite comfortable for some people.

If you go to SecretstoMeditation.com you will find a video called *Secrets to Meditation / Sitting.* In it you will see me demonstrating many of the suggestions I have made in this chapter.

A few final points on how to sit. There is an added benefit to sitting in a cross-legged position if it is comfortable. It gives you a more compact feeling than if your legs are spread out or dangling down from a chair. That feeling of compactness can help you focus and thus add further harmony to your practice.

The benefit of feeling compact while meditating leads me to share another secret, which is to consider wrapping yourself in a shawl. I teach that meditation shawls can be magical. They envelop you, and comfort you, much like swaddling a baby calms and comforts it. A shawl will give you the feeling of being hugged – warm, comfortable, soothing and calm. The compact feeling of a shawl can also help eliminate distractions and allow you to focus on your practice. If you are spiritually inclined, you can consider yourself being hugged by the Divine.

The last issue is what to do with your hands. Hands should either be in your lap, with one hand over the other and thumbs gently touching, or on your knees. Intertwining your fingers in your lap may cut off the circulation to your fingers after a while. Touching the thumbs is another subtle example of compactness. On your knees the hands can either be up or down. Up is more open to receiving from the Divine while down is somewhat more compact. If you are familiar with *mudras,* the hand positions in yoga, I encourage you to use one of them.

At our website SecretstoMeditation.com you will find a video called *Secrets to Meditation / Hand Positions (Mudras)*. In it I teach you how to feel the power and understand the symbolism contained in mudras. Your hands are sensitive and powerful tools. The position you choose can add even more meaning and harmony to your *Meditation Plus* practice.

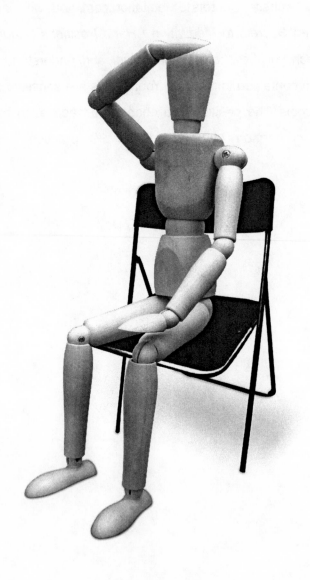

Let's turn to where to sit, which may be determined by how you're planning to sit. If you choose to meditate in bed or in your favorite cushy chair, where you meditate will be a given. But remember: You can meditate anywhere.

I have meditated in Grand Central Station, on airplanes, at the beach, in churches, temples and hospital waiting rooms. You name it, you can meditate there.

It's nice, however, to have a home base for your meditation. Again, this can be in your favorite chair or your bed. But if you can sit on the floor, or if you can move that favorite chair, then I highly recommend that you establish a special place, somewhere quiet, which you can make your sacred space. To make it feel sacred, you can set up an altar with religious symbols. You can place photos of loved ones there. If you have had inspiring teachers or spiritual mentors, you can add their pictures. You can decorate your space with fresh flowers or inspiring art work. You can burn incense or candles while you meditate. You can play soft music which might help drown out noises from traffic or others in your house.

The power of making a place special for meditating is its ability to produce a conditioned response in you whenever you sit there to meditate. Your body and mind expect to meditate there, expect to experience peace there, which will make it easier to settle into those states. Once again, however, this business of sacred space is optional, because ultimately, the sacredness – like the "teacher" – is found inside yourself.

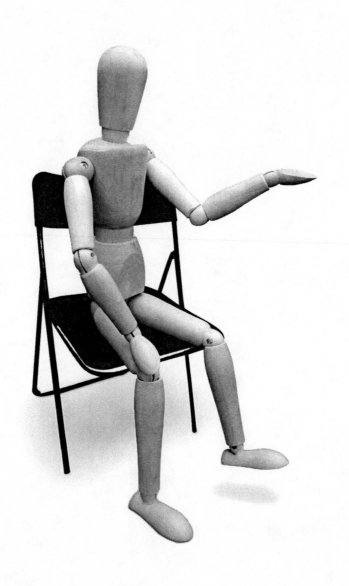

When to Sit

The third of the how, where and when questions is: When to sit and meditate? Again, the answer is personal and flexible. Meditate anytime you can.

There is a related issue I want to address along with when. How long to meditate? And I'm tempted to answer this question the same way. Meditate as long as is comfortable – comfortable both physically and within the context of your life, your work and your responsibilities.

Now that I have the glib answers out of the way, let's examine the challenges. I believe that if you really want to establish a meditation practice and reap its powerful benefits, it is important to meditate for at least 10 minutes every day. That 10 minutes of meditation every single day will give you 10 minutes of peace, every single day – 10 minutes of harmony, every single day – 10 minutes of clarity, every single day. It will add up to 60 hours of peace, harmony, and clarity each year. Over the years it will add up into hundreds and even thousands of hours of peace, harmony and clarity in your life.

The first line in my book, *Small Change; It's the Little Things in Life that Make a BIG Difference*, is that small change adds up. Put coins in a jar everyday, and watch them add up. Make small changes in your life, in your diet and exercise, in your work, in your relationships, in your leisure pursuits or in your spiritual practices, and watch them add up as well. Small change and small changes add up. Over time they can make a huge difference in your life. Meditating 10 minutes everyday is one of them.

Here's another analogy, both for meditation and the concept of change adding up. If you have a jar of dirty water, what is the best way to remove the dirt? Do you try to remove each small piece one at a time? Do you pour it through a filter into another container? Both can help but chances are, some dirt will remain.

Your life is like that jar of dirty water. Bad things have happened to all of us. Do you go into psychotherapy and examine each issue in an attempt to remove it, or get beyond it? Do you dramatically change your circumstances in an attempt to get over them? Both can help but chances are, some problems will still be there.

Meditation is the process of adding clear water. Everyday you sit and add 10 minutes of clarity. Will the "dirt" still be there? Of course, but over time, the dirt will be lost in an ocean of clarity. Add clarity to your life by meditating every single day. Watch your clarity add up and your problems subside.

Later in this book, I will try to convince you to meditate for 20 minutes each day – by adding 10 minutes of "clear thinking" after your 10 minutes of structured meditation. Yes, you read me correctly. I am a meditation teacher who will try to convince you to actually *think* during the time you set aside for meditation. But I can assure you that 10 minutes of "clear thinking" following your formal meditation practice will prove to be *the most productive thinking you do in your life*. It is one of the biggest pluses that this *Meditation Plus* technique has to offer, making it so much more effective. Because this thinking is often so profound, I encourage my students to keep a pen and pad of paper available for taking notes. Trust me. After learning to meditate, you will want to take the extra 10 minutes to think. For now though, just keep that option in the back of your mind.

We're looking for 10 to 20 minutes each day. (Notice how I snuck in those extra minutes.) Finding this time can be a challenge at first, especially if you are leading one of the typical, busy, 24/7 lives so many of us are coping with. So start with the minimum. Find 10 minutes. For most people, the easiest and best time is first thing in the morning, just after waking up and perhaps going to the bathroom, before your day gets hectic. Your home is often the most peaceful then, especially if you're the first one to wake up. You haven't eaten, which is considered an advantage, though not totally necessary. Many find that if you eat before meditating, you may have to deal with distracting noises and discomfort caused by your stomach's digestive process. Still, if meditating after a meal is most convenient, go for it. It will be better than not meditating at all.

If you can't meditate in the morning, or if you would like to add a second meditation to your day, you may find that meditating in the afternoon or after work will help you calm down, unload the stress of your job, and prepare you for an evening alone or with family or friends. Or, you may meditate before going to sleep. Meditating can calm your mind and help you sleep. This can be especially helpful on nights when your mind is racing and you can't seem to fall asleep. Studies have shown that meditation can help people get to sleep easier and sleep more effectively. The only problem goes back to wanting to be alert for your meditation, which may be counter-productive right before bedtime. You decide.

Notice, each time of day has advantages and disadvantages. Choose the best time for you, but be aware that you do not have to limit yourself to meditating once a day. Some teachers encourage meditating at least twice a day, to experience all the benefits of meditation. My goal is to get you started. Experiment with each possibility and decide what's right for you.

Once you have chosen when to meditate, hold to that time each day, if possible. The routine itself adds power. Your body and mind will become conditioned to the schedule, as it has become conditioned to eating meals at the same time each day. The body expects it. The body gets ready for it in anticipation. Hunger is the body's desire for the food it is expecting. Meditating at a set time each day will develop a hunger in your mind for the peace it is expecting.

For those of you convinced that you cannot find 10 minutes for meditation, let's return to the issue of sleep. My unabashed goal is to convince you that 10 minutes of meditation is better for you than 10 minutes of sleep, and that it would be worth getting up 10 minutes earlier each day. I know that might be a challenge, but allow me to try.

First, sleep is not always a restful state, while meditation is. Sleep experts claim that the body needs an average of two to three hours of deep sleep per night. The rest of your sleeping is spent in a combination of light sleep and REM (Rapid Eye Movement) or dream state. There is no substitute for deep sleep, which the body needs for replenishment. In contrast, the dream state is variable. Its purpose is to nurture and restore both your mental and emotional systems. Our dreams help us grapple with problems and the tension in our lives. We use symbols, recurring themes, and often disturbing circumstances to work through our frustrations. Our dreams can be frightening, exhilarating, frustrating or enjoyable. We need our dreams. Many experts say that four to six hours of light sleep and REM, added to the three hours of deep sleep, creates the ideal seven to nine hours of sleep needed for good health and emotional balance.

Here's my thinking: Trade 10 minutes of dreaming for 10 minutes of meditation. Why? Because studies are confirming that meditation is more relaxing and more efficient at calming your mind and emotions. Here's something to think about. During sleep, oxygen consumption in the body decreases slowly until, after about five hours, it reaches a level approximately 8% lower than wakefulness, a measure of your relaxation. In contrast, during meditation, oxygen consumption decreases to between 10% and 20% lower than wakefulness, and occurs within three minutes. Yes, after only three minutes of meditation your body is virtually twice as relaxed as after five hours of sleep!

So yes, I urge you to get up 10 minutes earlier to meditate. Now, I know that while this may sound reasonable, you may think differently when your alarm clock goes off, and 10 more minutes of sleep is so tempting. You will just have to power through that temptation. If you try this, I believe you will feel the benefits almost immediately. You will feel fresher, clearer, calmer and more ready for your day than sleeping that extra 10 minutes.

I'll close with my *Meditator's Rule of Thumb.* This is not a scientifically-based claim, although there is some research to support it, and I personally attest to its validity. Here it is:

Ten minutes of meditation = one hour of sleep.

I have tested this formula in a number of ways. Many years ago I went on what I called a "sleep-fast." I wanted to see how well I could function on only three hours of deep sleep each night. By the second night, when my body did not get enough deep sleep the night before, it began to grab its deep sleep first, allowing me to replace four to six hours of light sleep and REM with at least one hour of meditation. I would spend the rest of my night reading, doing yoga or working on the computer. That gave me an extra three to five hours of productive time each day. I promised myself that if I felt sleepy driving home from work at 5:30pm, I would pull off the road to rest and abandon my experiment. Here were the results.

I "sleep-fasted" for three full months. I never had to pull off the road coming home from work. As someone capable of sleeping around the clock at the time, I was amazed.

I also learned, however, how enjoyable sleep can be. Many of us say that we would like more hours in our day. The biggest issue with those extra hours was the potential for boredom. No one else was there to keep me company. Those books I wanted to read needed to be better than the lure of an enticing dream. I chose to break up that time with three 20-minute meditations rather than one 60-minute sitting. I could always count on the meditation to refresh me when a boring book was putting me to sleep.

I learned I needed to fuel those extra waking hours with more food. I added a fourth meal at about 11pm. Some current research shows that getting adequate sleep can help weight loss. I believe it. As long as my extra waking hours included added exercise, which for me was yoga, I was able to burn off the extra calories I was eating.

After three months, I chose to return to my usual pattern. I had learned that for me, a balance of REM and meditation felt right, and scientific research is confirming that conclusion. They are discovering that meditation clearly enhances the effectiveness of sleep, but should not be used as a substitute. I'm not encouraging you to follow me in a sleep fast, or to take the rule of thumb beyond the one hour. Besides, everyone is different. The real conclusion here is that meditation will help you find the right amount of sleep for you to function with optimum health and efficiency.

Meanwhile, there are still more practical benefits to understanding the relationship between meditation and sleep than just my argument that it's worth getting up 10 to 20 minutes earlier to meditate. Studies show that when subjects are tired and some are given a short nap, a period of relaxation or meditation, the meditators significantly out-perform the others on a test of alertness afterwards. So, if you are behind the wheel of your car and get tired, pulling off the road to meditate could be your safest and most efficient solution.

I also use meditation when I'm traveling through multiple time zones. I use the formula to calculate when and how long to meditate so that I can arrive in synch with my new surroundings.

I close this chapter with this caveat. Your experience with meditation will not be exactly the same as mine. Let your meditation be your guide. Experiment to find what is right for you. Trust yourself and trust your meditation.

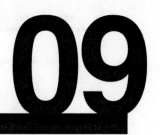
09

Finally, we're ready to begin meditating. Start with relaxation. As you have learned, your breath has two syllables, an inhale and an exhale. The inhale is the acquisition side. We inhale the oxygen that allows combustion to take place within every cell of our body. We inhale energy. We inhale life.

The exhale is the letting-go side of the breath. The exhale releases the carbon dioxide that is a product of that combustion. Your exhale cleanses, purifies and releases waste. While you're at it you might as well exhale some emotional waste as well. Use that exhale to let go of tension, stress, fear, anxiety, blame, judgment and even pain.

Use your exhale to relax. There are many techniques for doing this. You can tense and then relax your muscles, either progressively (legs first, then hands and arms, then stomach, then shoulders and then face) or tense and relax your entire body all at once. First inhale and squeeze the muscles while holding your breath, then exhale and let the muscles go totally limp.

You can also relax without tensing your muscles by turning your attention to each part of your body and feeling it relax with a conscious exhale. You can even use the two-syllable mantra, *re-lax,* to do this. On the inhale hear *re,* on the exhale hear a long, slow *lax,* as you feel and visualize the tension leaving your muscles, either progressively or all at once.

At the very least, take a few breaths to isolate and release tension from three specific areas – stomach, shoulders and face, because these are the three areas in your body that store the most tension. We routinely take our problems there. We tie our stomachs into knots. We hold our shoulders up towards our earlobes instead of relaxing them and letting them rest on the upper shelf of the ribcage. We tense up our face and our wrinkles deepen, reflecting the stress in our lives.

I have a personal theory about the tension we hold in our stomachs, shoulders and faces. I'm not claiming that it has been scientifically proven but it is an insight that has been very helpful to me and many of my students. I believe that much of the tension found in your stomach relates to the future. You take your worry into your stomach. You hold on to expectations, there. You try to get others to do what you want, from there. You resist change, there. When you relax your stomach, you open possibilities for the future. By relaxing your stomach you can transform fear into confidence, into trusting that good things will happen without your having to control every element of the process. So relax your stomach, and you will be relaxing into the rest of your life.

I believe that tension in your shoulders is primarily related to the past. Holding your shoulders up with tension is like lugging around an emotional backpack of everything that has happened to you. It is full of blame, shame, mistakes – yours or others – and all the things that others have done to you. It is your bag of excuses, your claim to the title of "victim." Dare to set it down. Leave the past in the past. You can't change it but you can change the hold it has on you. Give yourself credit for having survived. Relax the tension in your shoulders, and move forward lighter and freer.

Finally, I find that tension in your face seems to relate to the present moment. When you like what you are seeing or feeling, you tend to smile. When you don't like it, you frown or grimace. Your face reflects your present feelings. When your face is calm and smooth, like a still pond, the present moment is reflected exactly as it is, in all its glory. When that pond is agitated and disturbed, the reflection is unrecognizable. Strive to be that calm, serene, still pond. Smooth out your face, and receive the present as the gift that it is, savoring the miracle that you are experiencing.

To prepare for meditation, it's important to take the time you need to untie the knots in your stomach, release the tension in your shoulders and smooth out your face. Feel yourself coming into harmony with the future, the past and the present.

Next, we turn to your tongue – yes, your tongue. It is one of the strongest muscles in your body. I like to add that when used inappropriately, it can be the most dangerous muscle as well. It's important to relax it along with your other muscles. The tip of the tongue should rest gently behind the back of the upper front teeth. The sides and top of the tongue relax in gentle contact with the upper palate. The base of the tongue, down in the back of the throat where the tongue meets the windpipe, relaxes into what I like to visualize as an "inner smile."

The inner smile is a powerful secret skill with the ability to put you and your meditation into perspective. That smile keeps you from taking yourself or your practice too seriously. It helps put your thoughts into perspective. They are, after all, just thoughts. Smiling reduces their power. It sets you up as a witness, a curious spectator to your inner and outer worlds. It brings a level of detachment that helps prevent outside distractions from becoming annoying. The inner smile helps cultivate the mindfulness that Buddhist meditation practices strive for. I personally feel like I am smiling with the Divine, in on a cosmic joke that goes something like this: I came here to be me in this life. I understand that I don't get to be anyone else even though I might want to be. Why me? Because everyone else is taken!

Cultivating your secret inner smile, along with your meditation practice, will give you powerful tools to deal with the many mistakes we all make, along with the mistakes of others. Finding your inner smile helps you maintain a sense of humor while dealing with yourself, while dealing with others, and while dealing with the mysteries the Divine seems to present. It's a great way to approach many of the difficult issues in your life. As I like to say, "It is always better to smile with God than to cry alone."

After you have relaxed and found your inner smile, you are ready to begin "listening." Listen to the sound of your breath. Listen to the audible, two-syllable message it whispers. It provides a two-syllable vibration for tuning your mind and with it, your life.

This is the two-syllable mantra we discussed in Chapter Five. Many possible mantras were discussed there and more are listed at the back of this book. Which message do you hear? What vibration, what ability do you need to develop in your life? Do not limit yourself to the list provided. Trust your breath. Trust your feelings and your judgment. You know what you need. Tune into it.

I recommend that you define the technique of meditation as a duet between your mind and your breath. Your breath speaks ever so subtly and your mind joins internally in harmony with your breath. Both mind and breath are expressing the same word or phrase, the same message, the same vibration, the same mantra.

The next step is the shift we discussed in Chapter Two, in which the process changes from just thinking into witnessing what you are thinking, witnessing the duet, adding the mindfulness. Even though your mind is busy repeating your mantra, you can simultaneously become aware of that process, aware of that thinking. It is that awareness, even more than the repetition of the mantra itself, that is meditation. When you are enjoying the duet, as both a participant and a witness, at the same time, you are truly meditating.

Remember, the inner smile can facilitate that witnessing, that mindfulness. When I say enjoy the duet, one way to establish that enjoyment is by activating your inner smile at the base of the tongue, as if to say, "Look at this. I am thinking, in harmony with my breath, a special word, and I am aware of that process at the same time. How cool is that?" Even when random thoughts try to interfere, your ability to smile and witness those thoughts as just thoughts, maintains the continuity of your meditation. Don't forget. Meditation is not about not thinking. Meditation is found in the *relationship* we develop with our thinking. The duet technique, aided by the inner smile, facilitates that witnessing, mindful relationship.

Another secret technique for bringing energy and joy to your meditation is to put your duet into a swinging motion. Remember, using a swing is the easy way to levitate. As the inhale begins to form the first syllable of your mantra, experience the inhale as the backswing of your swing. Then, as the exhale begins forming the second syllable, feel that exhale as an exhilarating swing forward. Feel the letting go as you fly forward and up. Feel the "wheeee."

Enjoy the same emotions you had as a child swinging on a swing. Go back to that time, perhaps to the swing in your backyard or school playground. Do this consciously, aware of the process as you are doing it. Become a witness to your mind at all levels.

I want to give you one more secret trick. I call it kicking the duet, the swing, the conscious focus into a "higher gear." I call it that because in 2003, I volunteered to have my brainwaves projected on a screen, while meditating, at a major holistic health conference. A series of wires were attached to my skull to detect colored patterns of brain activity that changed with my thoughts and feelings. There were hundreds of people in the audience, and I had no idea what to expect.

I began my meditation process with relaxation, and I could hear the speaker explaining the pattern that began appearing on the screen. Then, as I listened to my breath and began the duet and the swing, the speaker explained how the pattern had morphed into what he called the classic meditation pattern. I was able to handle the external distraction of his voice the same way I approach the duet and any other thoughts that come up while meditating. I witness them, smile at them, and gently return to my duet and swing.

Next, as is my practice, once I establish the duet and swing, I gently focus my closed eyes and gaze up to my "third eye," the spot above my eyebrows in the middle of my forehead. Although my eyes do cross and look up in the process, I try not to make it stressful, just a gentle focusing, a gentle relocation of the duet and swing to that spot, a gentle gazing to go along with the inner smile and the witnessing. I'll talk about why I gaze at my forehead and not somewhere else in a moment, but let's return to my story.

As I gently focused, I could hear a loud gasp go through the audience. The pattern on the screen had become even clearer, and the colors had intensified throughout. The speaker could only say, "Wow. *That's* meditation." Later, he told me it was the strongest and most dramatic presentation of the brain in meditation he had ever seen.

The reason I'm sharing this story is to explain why I call the gentle focusing of the eyes to a spot inside your body "kicking your meditation into a higher gear." Eastern philosophy teaches that you have energy centers in your body called *chakras.* The body's four higher chakras – higher energy centers, higher levels of consciousness – are found in your heart, your throat, your forehead and the center of the top of your head. Your heart chakra vibrates love, your throat chakra vibrates happiness (note the location here of the inner smile), your forehead or third-eye chakra vibrates wisdom and your crown chakra, at the center of the top of your head, vibrates spirituality.

In your meditation practice, after you have relaxed and begun to enjoy the duet and the swing, make a conscious decision to take that duet and swing to one of those four chakras, one of your higher energy centers. You will either be gently gazing down to focus your duet at your heart or throat, or gazing up at your forehead or top of your head. Don't lift or lower your head. This is done with closed eyes, gently.

This gentle crossing of the eyes to gaze inside, at the chakra you choose, adds focus, and adds another level to your witnessing and to your harmony. Don't just believe me, try it. Add the gentle focusing and the vibrational energy of the chakras to your practice, and you will understand what I mean by "kicking your meditation into a higher gear."

Common questions I am asked when I teach meditation are, "How do I deal with the thoughts that keep interrupting my practice? My mind just won't quit."

Or, "What should I do about distractions that come up, such as police sirens, phones ringing or other people talking?" Still another is, "What should I do about physical discomfort, such as legs falling asleep or the need to sneeze or scratch an itch?"

One answer, which I described earlier, is to see the distractions as amusing. Return to the teaching of the "inner smile." It's amusing when the mind won't stop throwing out thoughts and ideas. It's amusing that the world seems determined to interrupt your practice with phone calls or birds chirping. And it's amusing that the body complains just when you want it to cooperate and let you meditate. See the humor there? It's not a conspiracy to keep you from meditating. It's who we are and the world we live in. Smile at it.

So, acknowledge the distractions, smile at them, take care of anything necessary to make you comfortable, and return to your meditation. If you were swinging on a swing, and a friend came over to say something to you, or if you had to tie a shoelace, you would simply stop swinging for a moment, take care of it and begin swinging again. I doubt if you would dwell on the fact that you had to stop swinging. Meditation swings can be the same.

Another related distraction is wondering what time it is. Perhaps you have to get to work or an appointment and you begin worrying that your meditation will cause you to be late. I keep a small digital clock where I meditate for just this problem. When the thought comes that I wonder how much time has gone by, I simply check the clock, smile and return to my practice. It's just a clock, it's not passing judgment. Be gentle while you work within any necessary time constraints.

Once again, the idea is not to let anything be too big a deal. If you have an itch, scratch it, then return to swinging with your breath. If you are uncomfortable, adjust your body or seat, then return to your duet. When thoughts interfere, acknowledge them, witness them, smile at them, then return to your mantra.

Remember, your mind is a gift, an incredible tool for generating thoughts and ideas. Before you get annoyed with it, be sure to honor it. Smiling at its thought-generating ability is a great way to honor the incredible job that your mind does for you.

Here's another secret for dealing with an uncooperative mind. Negotiate with it. Yes, negotiate with your mind. It goes like this. "Mind, I know you have thoughts and ideas to present to me, but could you *please* hold off for 10 minutes? I promise to let you present those ideas soon, but for now, please let me enjoy my duet, my swing… for a few more minutes?"

I have found that my mind can be like a small child. It wants to be heard…now. So it helps to buy a little time. Tell your mind you will be ready to deal with it in less than 10 minutes. Teach your mind a lesson in patience.

Here's the key. It is important to follow through on your promise. Live up to your end of the bargain – either with a small child or your mind. If you renege, that child will learn not to trust you. The child will throw a tantrum instead of patiently waiting. Minds are the same. Be a person of your word and leave some time to indulge your mind's desires.

This promise to pay attention to your mind after the formal meditation practice leads to one of the most powerful teachings of my meditation technique, and one of the biggest reasons my students call it *Meditation Plus*. You get the opportunity to think. Some meditation teachers would regard this idea – to indulge in thinking – as outrageous, because they teach that meditation is about *not* thinking. I say that one of the most powerful benefits of a meditation practice is that it gives you the ability to think clearly, to see your problems and potential solutions with a fresh perspective. Why not take advantage of that benefit?

How do you do that? You wait until after your 10 minutes of mindful, mantra meditation before turning to your thoughts and problems. As an analogy, you can see much clearer through a window after you have cleaned it. Your meditation, even for just 10 minutes, has the power to clean the window of your mind. Meditation clears away the conditioned responses you have used in the past. It frees you to look at issues differently. It opens up new choices, new options, new possibilities.

Here's an example. You have just had a fight with someone close to you and are extremely frustrated. Hey, you know you are right. Why doesn't the other person know you're right? Perhaps you thought raising your voice would dramatize your point but he/she still wasn't convinced. And now you seem to have no options left. You're right. The other person is wrong. That's all there is to it. Been there? Who hasn't?

When you sit down to meditate after an argument, your mind will usually start with "knowing" how right you were. After doing the practice, however, even for as little as 10 minutes, a number of things will happen. The relaxation starts to release some of the frustration you are feeling. The duet and swing tune you into the vibration of the mantra. The inner smile enables you to see, with amusement, the shortcomings of your own behavior, as well as the other person's. Then, when the window is clean, when you have more clarity, you can begin to explore possible solutions. You will see options that were not visible in the heat of the argument, and may not have become visible without meditation. You may realize that perhaps you weren't totally right after all, and that one option is apologizing.

Forgiveness is another possibility that might not have crossed your mind earlier. You could offer a hug of reconciliation and say, "I may not agree with you, but I do love you."

Meditation, and the calm reflection that follows, can produce options and even solutions. It helps you think clearly. Why not spend some time as part of your practice taking advantage of this opportunity? I guarantee that you will find this the most immediate benefit of meditating. In addition to settling our marital disputes, my wife and I have written all of our books from ideas that arose after meditating. We keep a pad of paper and pen nearby. Trust me. There will be many times when you will want to take notes.

My final point here is to remind you that negotiating with your mind is a powerful strategy to get it to give you the time you want and need to meditate. If you ask, your mind will give you that time. By taking time to think about your problems after meditating, you will be training your mind to know that it will get time to present its ideas, and that those ideas will be some of its best. You will become more committed to your practice when you see that your life benefits from the ideas you get. And your mind will learn to trust your offer to wait a few minutes before it gets its turn to indulge.

To ensure that you reap the full benefit from the time you have devoted to meditation, follow it up with these steps. First, with your eyes still closed, take a deep breath, then swallow. These two gentle actions signal your body and your mind that a transition is taking place – from meditation to the real world.

The deep breath brings you the energy you need to begin the transition out of meditation and on to the rest of your day. The swallow signals that the "meal" is over.

Next, it's nice to gently lower your chin, and silently invoke a prayer. It can be from a religious tradition, or you can wing it. You can address it to the Divine, or simply to the world itself. It can express your gratitude for the blessings you have received. You can ask for help and healing, or send help and healing to someone else. You can feel Divine light and love pouring over your head and shoulders, and you can share that light with people dear to you. You can visualize yourself encased in a bubble of white light that protects you, guides you and heals you. You can visualize those you love protected by that light as well. Then, bring your hands together into a prayer position at your heart, and express your gratitude by saying or thinking, "amen."

Slowly open your eyes. Consider this a magical moment, as if you are looking at your surroundings for the very first time. After meditation everything around you seems different, much clearer, truly amazing. The world seems to present itself with a freshness that wasn't there when you sat down to meditate. It may feel as if you have cleaned your window to the world and now the world appears so much brighter. Savor this amazement and enjoy it for as long as you can.

I like to teach that meditation, along with yoga, offers three gifts everytime you finish your practice. The first gift is gratitude. You feel grateful for the incredible body and mind you have been given, grateful for the wonderful people in your life, grateful for all you have been given – materially, emotionally and spiritually – to enjoy in this lifetime.

The second gift is amazement. When you come out of meditation or have finished a yoga session, you emerge with a fresh sense of wonder – for how amazing bodies and minds can be, for how amazing the world in which we live can be. Wow, it's amazing we ever got to be here at all! Yet here we are, in this amazing place, full of amazing people, with an amazing abundance of food, clothes, water and warmth.

This gift of amazement and wonder is how yoga and meditation earned the reputation for getting you high without drugs. It's in the amazement. I know I sound like a Sixties stoner, which I wasn't, but it is a similar experience and costs nothing. It is also legal, available everywhere, healthy and safe. Incidentally, the word "stoned" comes from the same root word as "astonished". Enjoy that astonishment when you open your eyes. Enjoy that amazement, that sense of wonder. It is the sense of awe that prophets and spiritual seekers experience and promote. I like to call it the *Twin Peaks* – a *peek* into how life can really be, a *peak* experience that life offers.

The third gift meditation offers is a sense of grace. Grace is the feeling of having received something special. Few people get to experience the glimpse into their own minds and being that meditation offers. Few take the time to explore this dimension of life. Few experience the consciousness that medittion brings. After meditating you feel as if you were chosen to receive a special gift. Feeling special, feeling chosen is what grace is about. To walk in grace is to live with the awareness of how special you are. In a religious context it is the awareness of how special you are in God's eyes, chosen to receive God's love. It reinforces both the gratitude and the amazement.

Gratitude, amazement and grace – three gifts you can take with you into your day and into your life. Hold on to these gifts and take them with you to your work, to your meals, to the time you spend with family and friends.

Some advice here. Don't feel the need to publicize what you're feeling. You don't need to brag about it. Nor do you need to explain it. You will know, and others will sense, that in a profound way you are different – more appreciative, more aware, more present, more at peace. An inner light will be glowing in you and will remain lit, fueled by your meditation and its gifts. Gratitude, amazement and grace provide the source for that light. Nurture those gifts, and watch them light up your life.

Tuning Back In

I want to share with you one final benefit of this specific meditation technique, one more *plus.* When you cultivate a mantra – along with its message and vibration – through daily practice, you can tune back into that mantra at anytime during the day.

When you feel stressed, when you have a difficult decision to make, when someone gives you a hard time, your mantra is only one breath away. Remember, your breath whispers its message to you approximately 20,000 times a day!

A consistent meditation practice will allow you to tap into the power of your mantra whenever you need it. I think of it as putting the world on my side, feeling and hearing it cheering me on. I think of it as having the Divine as my companion, always there to remind me, encourage me, coach me to achieve what I have set out to accomplish.

"Take a deep breath." We have all received this advice. When we are stressed out, we should take a deep breath. *Meditation Plus* takes this teaching a step farther. Taking a breath will not just calm your nerves. Your breath will actually speak to you, calling for you to "re-tune" your instrument. Your breath has the power to bring you back into harmony with the music of your life.

Meditation Plus also develops your ability to tune in, at will, to the "inner smile" at the back of your throat. You can use that smile to witness your thoughts throughout your day, and put those thoughts into perspective. Smiling can ease even the most stressful situations. We can see the humor in our mistakes and that we can learn from those mistakes.

We all know that life is not always fair. In school, we complain when a test includes questions on material not covered in class. In life, however, we are routinely tested first, and only *after* the test do we get the teachings. Once you understand that, you can smile. It's another one of the cosmic jokes that you will have understood.

I often think of a pessimistic old Jewish saying, which reflects the strength of a people who have suffered greatly throughout history. "People make plans and God laughs." I like to put a different spin on its teaching, repeating the maxim I referred to earlier. "It is better to laugh with God than to cry alone."

The inner smile you cultivate in meditation reminds you that you can transcend your body and your mind. It reminds you that you have the ability to witness your thoughts from an enjoyable perspective. I like to consider that inner smile a "cosmic smile," for it is a smile you can share with the Divine, as if you and the Divine are in on the cosmic jokes together. Yes God, I get it. Everyone else is taken.

When it comes to speculating on why we are here, in this life, many preach about a Judgment Day or the Hereafter. This much I know. We are here, on this planet, in this life, to learn. We know more today than we knew yesterday. We know more than we knew five years ago. Of course, many of us would like to go back, to be young again. But we only want to go back with the wisdom and knowledge we have gained in the years since.

Life is about learning. We learn about ourselves, about others, about the world we live in. We learn what's important and what isn't. We learn about love. Once we understand that we are here to learn, once we get it, we can smile. Sometimes we sleep-walk through life, following routines as if on autopilot. The world has to hit us over the head with two-by-fours to get our attention. The mantra, whispered by the breath, is our gentle, on-going call to wake up, to listen, to observe, to learn and to smile.

In Chapter Two I described my experience with the mantra OM, an experience that taught me I did not want a meditation practice that took me away from this world. Nor did I want to meditate just for the sake of meditation, just to feel good while I was doing it. I wanted a practice that would help me understand – and succeed – in the world I live in. I wanted a practice that would give me joy beyond the 20 minutes of my meditation. I wanted a practice that would enrich me on all levels – physically, mentally, emotionally and spiritually. I wanted a practice that would deepen my relationships – with myself, with my family, with my community, with the Divine.

I have found all of that in the *Meditation Plus* practice I have described. I can't imagine starting a day without meditation. I have meditated daily for over 40 years, and it has made my life truly magical. I believe, wholeheartedly, that *Meditation Plus* can do the same for you. But you have to give it a chance. Meditation takes time, commitment and follow-through. I am convinced that if you make the investment, the time you spend in meditation will pay dividends in every area of your life.

I invite you to join me as a fellow meditator. I invite you to see for yourself how easy and how powerful a meditation practice can be. You will get in tune with yourself, your life and the lives of the people you care about. Everyone – you, the people in your life and, in the process, the world – will benefit.

My prayer for you is that you will find the harmony you seek, along with the health, the love, the prosperity and the happiness that you are in this world to experience. Enjoy your meditation practice, and

Enjoy your journey!

1. **Place:** You can meditate anywhere, but it helps to have a special place. An altar with pictures, flowers, incense, candles or soft music is optional, but will make your space feel sacred. Eliminate as many distractions as possible, such as a phone or TV.

2. **Posture:** Sit comfortably and alert, with as straight a spine as possible. Your lumbar curve should be in its natural, inverted position, allowing your chest to remain open. If you sit on the floor in a cross-legged position, use a pillow under your buttocks to help support your lumbar curve and spine. (I even use a small pillow in lotus.) If you meditate in a chair or sit up in bed, use a pillow behind your lower back for lumbar support. On the chair you can sit on the forward edge, allowing the tilt of your pelvis to align your spine. Sitting cross- legged, if comfortable, makes you feel a little more compact, as does wrapping yourself in a special shawl.

   Your head should be balanced and unsupported, if possible. Your chin should be slightly drawn in, lifting your head, chest and spine. Hands can be in your lap, with one hand over the other and thumbs gently touching, or on your knees, palms up or down. If you are familiar with *mudras* – the hand positions in yoga – consider using one.

3. **Relaxation:** Begin by consciously relaxing the muscles of your body. You can use the tension/release technique, or use your exhale to carry away tension from your body. Pay particular attention to your stomach, shoulders and face. Release the tension in your stomach, and release your fears regarding the future. Release the tension in your shoulders, and release the grip of the past. Smooth out your face to reflect the present moment, clearly and beautifully.

4. **Focusing and Tuning:** Relax your tongue and throat and find your inner smile. Your tongue should touch the top of your palate, with the tip touching the back of your upper front teeth. Relax the base of the tongue, where the tongue meets the windpipe, and feel your breath pass through your inner smile there.

Become aware of the sound of your breath, the inhale and exhale. Listen for your mantra, gently audible in your breath's whisper. Form a duet with your mind and your breath. Consider invoking the image of a swing – pulling back with your inhale, flying forward and up on your exhale.

Kick your meditation into a higher gear by focusing your eyes on one of the higher *chakras.* Gaze down to your heart or throat, or up to your forehead or the top of your head. Take the duet, the sound, the vibration and the swing, to that *chakra* and, using your inner smile, enjoy them there for at least 10 minutes.

Don't make distractions a big deal. If tension builds in the body, notice the tension, exhale it away and return to your duet. If you have an itch, scratch it, and return to your mantra. If you need to check the time, glance at the clock, and return to your swinging. If you find yourself nodding off, bring your chin in to lift your head and spine. Don't make anything a big deal, just keep returning to the inner smile, to your duet, to your swing.

If thoughts come, don't allow them to become a big deal, either. Observe the thought, smile, and return to your duet. Or, negotiate with your mind. Ask it for 10 minutes to meditate, after which you will allow it to present its thoughts. Then, when you're ready, do exactly that. Ask your mind a question. Indulge in an imaginary conversation with yourself or someone else. Think about your problems, your options or what you are learning at this time in your life. Have pen and paper ready to take notes.

5. **Return to the World:** When you are ready to come out, take a deep breath and swallow.

Lower your head into a position of gratitude and humility, and invoke a prayer of your choice. Feel light and love surrounding you, protecting you, healing you, and share that light with others in your life. Bring your hands to your heart in prayer position, and close with "amen."

When you are ready, straighten up, become aware of your body, your senses, your feelings and your thoughts. Open your eyes. Look out at your surroundings as if you are seeing them for the first time. Observe your amazement. Acknowledge your gratitude. Feel the grace. Stretch out your body. Now carry that inner peace and consciousness with you as you get up and walk out into the rest of your day.

6. **Tune back in:** Throughout your day, catch moments when you hear your breath continuously whispering your mantra. Acknowledge its persistence with your inner smile. Hear its constant reminder to tune your body, your mind, your life to the message and vibration you know you need. Let it help you find the harmony that multiplies your effort, helping you swing higher in everything you do.

Enjoy your journey!

List of Mantras

Mantras are sounds, words or vibrations that serve as tuning forks for harmonizing your mind, your heart, your body and your life. They are the breath's whisper, reminding you what is important, and what you need to learn at this point in your life.

Practical English Mantras:

Loving	Healing	Wisdom
Relax	Let Go	Forgive
Happy	Worthy	Patience
I Can	I'm Strong	I Am
Focus	Courage	Power

Spiritual English Mantras:

Amen	Holy	Blessing
Divine	Spirit	God's Love

You can also use "now" or "wow" after a one-syllable word such as:
God, Peace, Love, Strength, Faith, Trust

Christian Mantras:

Jesus	God's Grace	Gospel
Mary	Savior	Heaven

Muslim Mantras:

Allah (God)   Salaam (Peace)

Koran (Divine Recitation)

Sanskrit Mantras:

So Hum

(I call this the "wow" mantra since it translates into "All that is... is."
Its vibration is amazement.)

Shanti (Peace)   Sat Nam (Truth is God's Name)

Satya (Truth)   Yoga (Union, Harmony)

Hindu Mantras:

Shiva   Rama   Kali

Krishna   Brahma   Shakti

Vishnu   Ganesh

(Hindu Gods/Goddesses representing qualities of the Divine.)

Buddhist Mantras:

Buddha (Enlightenment)   Dharma (Wisdom, Truth)

Hebrew Mantras:

Shalom (Peace)   YahWeh (The Secret Name of God)

Bracha (Blessing)   Chesed (Loving Kindness)

Torah (Divine Guidance)   Simcha (Happiness)

Echod (Oneness)   Shema (Listen and Hear)

Note that the above lists are not the only mantras you can use.

They are ones I have used and know to be effective. Decide what

your breath is whispering to you, and what vibration you need to

bring harmony into your life.

About the Author

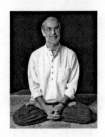

Larry Terkel received a B.S. in Industrial Engineering and an M.B.A., both from Cornell University. He also earned an M.A. in Philosophy and Comparative Religion from Kent State University. This dual pursuit of business and spirituality has continued throughout his professional career.

On the spiritual side, Larry was born Methodist, adopted by a Jewish family, is part Cherokee Indian, and spent extensive time studying Hinduism, Buddhism and yoga in India and throughout the world. In 1978, he acquired the Old Church on the Green in Hudson, Ohio, where he founded the Spiritual Life Society, one of northern Ohio's most unique spiritual centers. The Spiritual Life Society is an interdenominational organization that promotes the wisdom found within all religious traditions. Larry serves as the Society's minister and director, where he continues to teach yoga, meditation and philosophy on a regular basis.

Larry and his wife Susan are co-authors of the book, *Small Change; It's the Little Things in Life that Make a BIG Difference* (Tarcher/Penguin), a finalist for a Books for a Better Life Award. It was recommended by Jack Canfield *(Chicken*

Soup® series) and Barbara de Angeles, Ph.D. *(What Women Want Men to Know)* and acclaimed by *USA Today* as "How to Reach the Summit of Life's Success." *Small Change* provides insight into Larry and Susan's remarkable life together and presents their philosophy for self-improvement, based on bringing awareness to everyday habits. Married in 1970, they have three grown children and three grandchildren.

In his business career, Larry has been president of several companies, CEO of a public company and is currently president of Global HealthCare, Inc.

LARRY IS AVAILABLE FOR KEYNOTES, CONFERENCES, WORKSHOPS AND RETREATS.

SecretstoMeditation.com / MeditationPlus.net